DARREN COLE

The Science of Fat Loss

Dedication

To my beloved parents

Without your love, support, and encouragement, this book would not have been possible. Your unwavering belief in me has been a constant source of inspiration, and your sacrifices have allowed me to pursue my passion.

Contents

1.

2.

3.

4.

5.

6.

7.

8.

9.

10.

11.

12.

13.

Acknowledgement

I am deeply grateful to all the people who have helped and supported me in the writing of this book. First and foremost, I would like to thank my family for their unwavering love and encouragement, especially my partner who provided me with invaluable feedback and support throughout the entire process.

I would also like to express my heartfelt appreciation to my editor and the entire team at the publishing house for their hard work, patience, and support. Their insightful feedback and guidance were instrumental in shaping the final version of this book.

Furthermore, I am indebted to my friends and colleagues who have provided me with valuable insights, feedback, and inspiration along the way. Your encouragement and support have been a source of strength and motivation for me.

Finally, I would like to acknowledge the countless writers, scholars, and thinkers who have inspired me throughout my life. Their work has not only influenced my writing but has also enriched my worldview and perspective on the world.

Thank you all for being a part of this journey with me.

One

Introduction

A fat loss plan is a structured approach to losing body fat by creating a calorie deficit through a combination of diet and exercise. The goal of a fat loss plan is to reduce body fat while preserving lean muscle mass, and it typically involves setting a target weight loss goal, tracking food intake and exercise, and making lifestyle changes to support sustainable progress. An effective fat loss plan should be personalized to an individual's unique needs and preferences, and it should be based on sound nutrition principles and a safe and appropriate level of physical activity.

Two

When Fat Leaves The Body

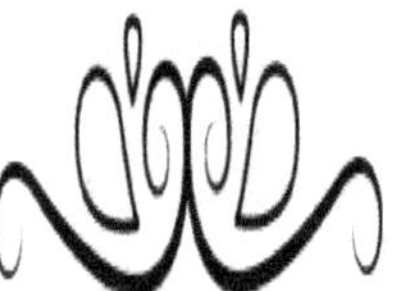

Fat loss pills are marketed as a way to help individuals lose weight quickly and easily. However, the safety of these pills has been a topic of much debate and concern.

Firstly, it's important to note that fat loss pills come in different types, including prescription medications and over-the-counter supplements. Prescription medications, such as orlistat, are FDA-approved and can help individuals lose weight when used under the supervision of a healthcare professional. However, they may have side effects such as oily stools, gas, and stomach cramping.

Over-the-counter fat loss supplements, on the other hand, are not regulated by the FDA, and their safety and effectiveness are not well-established. These supplements often contain a mix of herbs, vitamins, and other ingredients that are claimed to promote weight loss. However, the evidence supporting their use is limited, and some of these ingredients may have harmful side effects.

Furthermore, some fat loss pills can interact with other medications or medical conditions, which can be dangerous. For example, some fat loss pills can raise blood pressure or heart rate, which can be harmful for individuals with cardiovascular disease.

In general, it's important to consult with a healthcare professional before taking any fat loss pills or supplements. They can help you determine whether a particular product is safe and appropriate for you, and can provide guidance on how to use it effectively.

Overall, fat loss pills can be safe when used appropriately and under the guidance of a healthcare professional. However, it's important to be cautious and aware of the potential risks associated with these products, and to make informed decisions about their use.

Three

Fat Loss Diet Plan

Fat loss diets are designed to help individuals lose body fat while preserving lean muscle mass. The goal of these diets is to create a calorie deficit, which means consuming fewer calories than your body burns each day. This forces your body to use stored fat as fuel, leading to fat loss.

Here are some key components of a successful fat loss diet:

Calorie deficit: To lose fat, you need to be in a calorie deficit. This means consuming fewer calories than your body burns each day. A moderate calorie deficit of 300-500 calories per day is a good starting point.

Macronutrient balance: The macronutrients in your diet - protein, carbohydrates, and fat - all play important roles in fat loss. A balanced diet that includes enough protein to preserve muscle mass, complex carbohydrates for energy, and healthy fats for satiety is essential.

Protein: Adequate protein intake is crucial for fat loss. Protein helps preserve muscle mass while you're in a calorie deficit, and it also has a higher thermic effect than carbohydrates or fat, meaning your body burns more calories digesting it.

Complex carbohydrates: Carbohydrates are an important source of energy, but not all carbs are created equal. Complex carbohydrates, like whole grains and vegetables, provide sustained energy and fiber, which helps keep you feeling full and satisfied.

Healthy fats: Fat is an important macronutrient for overall health and satiety. Healthy sources of fat, like nuts, seeds, avocado, and olive oil, can help keep you feeling full and satisfied while in a calorie deficit.

Hydration: Staying hydrated is important for overall health and can also help with fat loss. Drinking plenty of water can help reduce feelings of hunger and may even help boost your metabolism.

Consistency: Consistency is key when it comes to fat loss. It's important to stick to your diet plan and make healthy choices every day, even on weekends and holidays.

In addition to following a healthy diet, incorporating regular exercise and getting enough sleep are also important for fat loss. Resistance training, in particular, can help preserve muscle mass while in a calorie deficit.

It's important to remember that fat loss takes time and patience. While rapid weight loss may be tempting, it's not sustainable in the long term and can lead to muscle loss and other negative health effects. Gradual, sustainable fat loss is the key to long-term success.

Four

What Fat Supplement Really Works

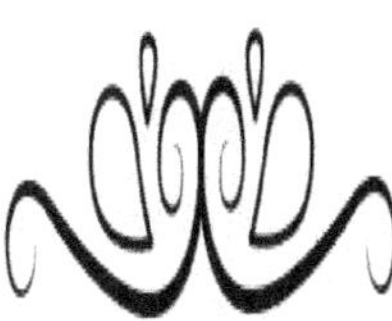

There are a variety of fat supplements on the market that claim to help people lose weight or burn fat more effectively. However, it is important to note that there is no magic pill or supplement that can replace a healthy diet and exercise regimen.

That being said, some fat supplements may provide some benefit when used in combination with a healthy lifestyle. Here are a few that have been studied:

Omega-3 Fatty Acids: Omega-3s are a type of healthy fat found in fish oil and some plant sources. Studies have shown that omega-3s may help reduce inflammation and improve insulin sensitivity, both of which may contribute to weight loss.

Conjugated Linoleic Acid (CLA): CLA is a type of fatty acid found in dairy products and beef. Some studies suggest that CLA may help reduce body fat and improve body composition.

Green Tea Extract: Green tea contains a compound called EGCG, which has been shown to increase fat oxidation and boost metabolism.

L-Carnitine: L-carnitine is an amino acid that helps transport fatty acids into cells to be burned for energy. Some studies suggest that L-carnitine may improve fat oxidation and reduce fatigue during exercise.

Fiber Supplements: Fiber supplements can help increase feelings of fullness and promote weight loss by slowing down the digestion and absorption of carbohydrates.

It is important to note that while these supplements may provide some benefit, they are not a substitute for a healthy diet and regular exercise. Additionally, it is always a good idea to talk to a healthcare professional before starting any new supplement regimen.

Five

Fat Loss Exercises

Fat loss exercises are physical activities that help to reduce body fat, improve fitness, and promote overall health. There are various forms of exercises that can contribute to fat loss, including cardiovascular exercises, strength training, and high-intensity interval training (HIIT).

Cardiovascular exercises, also known as aerobic exercises, are activities that increase heart rate and breathing rate. Examples of cardiovascular exercises include running, cycling, swimming, brisk walking, and jumping jacks. These types of exercises burn calories and help to reduce body fat. Cardiovascular exercises should be performed at least 3-5 times a week for 30-60 minutes per session to see significant fat loss.

Strength training exercises help to build and maintain lean muscle mass, which can increase metabolism and promote fat loss.

Examples of strength training exercises include weightlifting, resistance band workouts, and bodyweight exercises such as push-ups, squats, and lunges. Strength training exercises should be performed 2-3 times a week, with each session lasting 30-60 minutes.

HIIT workouts involve short bursts of high-intensity exercise followed by periods of rest or low-intensity exercise. HIIT workouts are effective in burning calories and reducing body fat due to their high-intensity nature. Examples of HIIT exercises include sprinting, jumping jacks, burpees, and mountain climbers. HIIT workouts can be performed 2-3 times a week, with each session lasting 20-30 minutes.

Incorporating a combination of cardiovascular exercises, strength training, and HIIT workouts into a fitness routine can help to maximize fat loss and improve overall health. It is important to also focus on a balanced and nutritious diet in conjunction with exercise to achieve optimal fat loss results.

Six

Are Fat Loss Piles Safe

Fat loss pills are marketed as a way to help individuals lose weight quickly and easily. However, the safety of these pills has been a topic of much debate and concern.

Firstly, it's important to note that fat loss pills come in different types, including prescription medications and over-the-counter supplements. Prescription medications, such as orlistat, are FDA-approved and can help individuals lose weight when used under the supervision of a healthcare professional. However, they may have side effects such as oily stools, gas, and stomach cramping.

Over-the-counter fat loss supplements, on the other hand, are not regulated by the FDA, and their safety and effectiveness are not well-established. These supplements often contain a mix of herbs, vitamins, and other ingredients that are claimed to promote weight loss. However, the evidence supporting their use is limited, and some of these ingredients may have harmful side effects.

Furthermore, some fat loss pills can interact with other medications or medical conditions, which can be dangerous. For example, some fat loss pills can raise blood pressure or heart rate, which can be harmful for individuals with cardiovascular disease.

In general, it's important to consult with a healthcare professional before taking any fat loss pills or supplements. They can help you determine whether a particular product is safe and appropriate for you, and can provide guidance on how to use it effectively.

Overall, fat loss pills can be safe when used appropriately and under the guidance of a healthcare professional. However, it's important to be cautious and aware of the potential risks associated with these products, and to make informed decisions about their use.

Mindset and Motivation

maintaining a healthy weight is essential for leading a healthy lifestyle. However, achieving fat loss can be a challenging task that requires discipline, dedication, and persistence. Mindset and motivation play a vital role in achieving fat loss goals.

Mindset refers to the attitudes and beliefs that individuals hold about themselves and their abilities. A growth mindset is an essential tool for successful weight loss. It involves viewing challenges as opportunities for growth and improvement. Individuals with a growth mindset understand that they can improve their abilities with effort, practice, and determination. In contrast, individuals with a fixed mindset believe that their abilities are set in stone, and they cannot improve them.

To achieve fat loss, individuals must adopt a growth mindset and embrace the challenge of making lifestyle changes. They should view setbacks and failures as opportunities to learn and adjust their approach. This approach allows individuals to develop healthy habits and maintain them over time.

Motivation is the driving force that propels individuals towards their goals. It is essential to stay motivated during the fat loss journey. There are two types of motivation: intrinsic and extrinsic. Intrinsic motivation comes from within and involves doing an activity for its inherent satisfaction. Extrinsic motivation comes from external rewards, such as money or recognition. While both types of motivation can be effective, intrinsic motivation is more sustainable in the long run.

To stay motivated during the fat loss journey, individuals should set specific and achievable goals. They should focus on the benefits of a healthy lifestyle, such as increased energy, improved mood, and reduced risk of chronic diseases. It is also essential to track progress and celebrate successes along the way.

In addition to mindset and motivation, there are other tools that individuals can use to achieve fat loss. These include:

Proper nutrition: A balanced diet that includes whole foods, lean protein, healthy fats, and complex carbohydrates can help individuals achieve fat loss.

Regular exercise: Physical activity can help individuals burn calories, build muscle, and improve their overall health.

Stress management: Chronic stress can lead to weight gain and hinder fat loss. Learning stress management techniques, such as meditation or deep breathing, can help individuals manage stress and achieve fat loss.

Sleep: Getting enough sleep is essential for weight management. Sleep deprivation can lead to hormonal imbalances that can hinder fat loss.

Mindset and motivation are essential tools for achieving fat loss. Individuals should adopt a growth mindset, set specific and achievable goals, and focus on the benefits of a healthy lifestyle. By combining these tools with proper nutrition, regular exercise, stress management, and adequate sleep, individuals can achieve their fat loss goals and maintain a healthy weight over time.

Eight

Fat Loss Plateau

Fat loss plateau refers to a situation where an individual stops losing weight despite maintaining a calorie deficit diet and exercise routine. It is a common phenomenon that people experience during their weight loss journey, and it can be frustrating and demotivating.

The human body is designed to maintain homeostasis, which means that it adapts to changes in the environment and tries to maintain a balance. When an individual starts to lose weight, the body tries to adapt by slowing down the metabolism, reducing the number of calories burned at rest, and increasing hunger and cravings for food. These adaptations make it challenging to continue losing weight.

There are several reasons why a person may experience a fat loss plateau, and some of the most common ones are:

Reduced Metabolic Rate: When an individual starts losing weight, the body's metabolism slows down to adjust to the calorie deficit. However, as the individual continues to lose weight, the body adapts to the new metabolic rate, and weight loss slows down.

Lack of Physical Activity: When an individual reduces their calorie intake to lose weight, they may also reduce their physical activity level, which can lead to a reduction in muscle mass and a slower metabolic rate.

Inadequate Calorie Deficit: An inadequate calorie deficit can lead to slow or no weight loss. It is essential to maintain a moderate calorie deficit of 300 to 500 calories per day to lose weight gradually.

Hormonal Imbalances: Hormonal imbalances, such as an underactive thyroid gland, can slow down the metabolic rate and make it challenging to lose weight.

Inconsistent Diet and Exercise: Inconsistent diet and exercise routines can also cause a fat loss plateau. It is crucial to maintain a consistent diet and exercise regimen to see consistent results.

To break through a fat loss plateau, an individual may need to make some changes to their diet and exercise routine. Here are some strategies that may help:

Increase Physical Activity: Increasing physical activity can help increase metabolism, burn more calories, and promote weight loss.

Modify Calorie Intake: Adjusting calorie intake can help to create a calorie deficit that will promote weight loss. It is essential to ensure that the calorie deficit is not too high, as this can lead to muscle loss and a slower metabolic rate.

Add Resistance Training: Resistance training can help to increase muscle mass, which can increase metabolism and promote weight loss.

Manage Stress: Stress can cause hormonal imbalances, which can slow down the metabolic rate and make it challenging to lose weight. Managing stress through techniques such as meditation, deep breathing, and yoga can help to promote weight loss.

Get Adequate Sleep: Lack of sleep can also cause hormonal imbalances, which can slow down the metabolic rate and make it challenging to lose weight. Getting adequate sleep can help to promote weight loss.

A fat loss plateau is a common phenomenon that people experience during their weight loss journey. It is essential to understand the reasons behind the plateau and make appropriate changes to the diet and exercise routine to break through it. With patience, persistence, and consistency, it is possible to achieve weight loss goals and maintain a healthy weight.

Nine

Sustainable Fat Loss

Sustainable fat loss is a long-term approach to weight loss that focuses on making lifestyle changes that can be maintained over time. The goal is to lose body fat while maintaining muscle mass, without relying on fad diets or extreme exercise regimens. Sustainable fat loss involves making small, gradual changes to one's diet and exercise habits, with the ultimate goal of creating a healthier, more balanced lifestyle.

The following are some key components of sustainable fat loss:

Caloric deficit: Sustainable fat loss requires that one consume fewer calories than they burn. This can be achieved through a combination of reducing caloric intake and increasing physical activity. However, it is important to ensure that the calorie deficit is not too severe, as this can lead to muscle loss and other negative health effects.

Balanced diet: Sustainable fat loss involves following a balanced diet that includes a variety of nutrient-dense foods. This means consuming plenty of fruits, vegetables, lean protein, and healthy fats, while limiting processed foods, sugary drinks, and other sources of empty calories.

Regular exercise: Sustainable fat loss requires regular physical activity, which can help burn calories, build muscle, and improve overall health. This can include a combination of cardio and strength training exercises, as well as other activities such as yoga or Pilates.

Adequate rest and recovery: Rest and recovery are important components of sustainable fat loss. This means getting enough sleep each night, allowing for rest days between workouts, and taking steps to manage stress, such as through meditation or other relaxation techniques.

Sustainable lifestyle changes: Sustainable fat loss involves making lifestyle changes that can be maintained over time. This may include developing healthy habits such as meal planning, cooking at home, and finding enjoyable forms of physical activity. It is important to find sustainable ways to incorporate healthy habits into one's daily routine, rather than relying on short-term solutions or quick fixes.

Sustainable fat loss is a holistic approach to weight loss that focuses on long-term health and well-being. By making small, gradual changes to one's diet and exercise habits, it is possible to achieve sustainable fat loss and maintain a healthy weight over time.

However, it is important to consult with a healthcare professional before starting any new diet or exercise program, especially if you have any underlying health conditions or concerns.

Ten

Physiology of Fat Loss

Fat loss, also known as weight loss, is a common goal for many individuals. The physiology of fat loss is complex, and involves multiple physiological systems and processes. In this note, we will discuss the key physiological factors involved in fat loss.

Metabolism

The process of metabolism is essential for fat loss. Metabolism refers to the chemical processes that occur within the body to maintain life. The rate of metabolism is influenced by several factors, including age, gender, body composition, and physical activity level.

When the body is in a state of negative energy balance, which means that it is burning more calories than it is consuming, it will begin to break down stored fat to use as energy. This process is known as lipolysis. The energy released from lipolysis can be used to fuel physical activity or other bodily processes.

Hormones

Hormones also play a key role in fat loss. Hormones are chemical messengers that are produced by the endocrine glands and are responsible for regulating many physiological processes, including metabolism and appetite.

The hormone insulin plays a particularly important role in fat loss. Insulin is produced by the pancreas in response to elevated blood glucose levels. Insulin promotes the storage of glucose in the liver and muscle tissue, and inhibits the breakdown of stored fat. Therefore, in order to promote fat loss, it is important to maintain low insulin levels.

Another important hormone in fat loss is leptin. Leptin is produced by adipose tissue and plays a role in regulating appetite and energy expenditure. When levels of leptin are low, appetite is increased and metabolism is decreased, which can lead to weight gain. Conversely, when leptin levels are high, appetite is suppressed and metabolism is increased, which can lead to weight loss.

Diet

Diet plays a critical role in fat loss. In order to lose fat, it is necessary to create a calorie deficit, which means that the body is burning more calories than it is consuming. This can be achieved through a combination of calorie restriction and increased physical activity.

In addition to calorie restriction, it is also important to consume a diet that is rich in nutrients and low in processed foods and refined sugars. Consuming a diet that is high in protein and fiber can help to increase feelings of fullness and reduce overall calorie intake.

Exercise

Exercise is another key factor in fat loss. Physical activity increases energy expenditure, which can help to create a calorie deficit and promote fat loss. In addition to increasing energy expenditure, exercise can also help to increase muscle mass, which can help to increase metabolism and promote fat loss.

In order to achieve optimal fat loss, it is recommended to engage in both cardio and resistance training exercises. Cardiovascular exercise, such as running or cycling, can help to increase energy expenditure and promote fat loss, while resistance training exercises, such as weight lifting, can help to increase muscle mass and promote a higher resting metabolic rate.

The physiology of fat loss is complex and involves multiple physiological systems and processes. To achieve optimal fat loss, it is important to focus on creating a calorie deficit through a combination of calorie restriction and increased physical activity, while also focusing on consuming a nutrient-rich diet and engaging in both cardio and resistance training exercises.

Eleven

Conclusion

In summary, fat reduction is a complex process that includes a calorie deficit, frequent exercise, and a well-balanced diet. While there are numerous approaches and strategies for achieving fat loss, it is critical to prioritize long-term sustainable and healthy habits. Consultation with a healthcare expert or a qualified dietician can assist individuals looking to embark on a fat loss journey with tailored counsel and support.

About the Author

Also by Darren Cole